LIVING WITH HIV

IN SELF & OTHERS

First published July 1988 by GMP Publishers Ltd,
P O Box 247, London N15 6RW

Distributed in North America by Alyson Publications Inc.,
40 Plympton St, Boston, MA 02118.

British Library Cataloguing in Publication Data

McMullen, Richie J.
Living with HIV in self and others.
1. Man. AIDS
I. Title
616.9'792

ISBN 0-85449-084-1

Illustrations by Derek Brazell
Printed in the European Community
by Norhaven A/S, Viborg, Denmark

LIVING WITH HIV

IN SELF & OTHERS

RICHIE McMULLEN

GMP

INTRODUCTION: LIVING WITH LIVING

This book is about living! It is for those who have the HIV disease and for those who haven't. It's for all those who wish to explore the vast inner resources of their own potential. It is NOT a how-to-live book, but rather a book in which I unashamedly and often subjectively expose my own vulnerabilities as a man with HIV disease.

HIV disease covers a wide and often confused spectrum, with AIDS being only a small part. When people speak of 'the AIDS virus' they are talking nonsense. The virus is HIV.

This book is about being fully human and fully alive!

LIVING WITH THE FACTS

Q. What do the letters 'H.I.V' actually stand for?

H = Human

I = Immunodeficiency

V = Virus

Q. What does the virus do?

The virus has an attraction, or affinity, for specialised white cells in the blood. These are called 'T-lymphocyte cells' and they play an important role in helping the body to fight infection. The HIV actually invades and lives inside these T-cells, ultimately destroying them.

Q. If I have the virus, does that mean I will get AIDS?

Not necessarily! A positive test result does mean that the person has been exposed to the virus but it does NOT necessarily mean that the person will develop AIDS.

People who get a positive test result, that is, they have the antibodies present, are known as 'seropositive' and do not necessarily develop AIDS. It is known that at present some 30% of those with HIV will go on to develop AIDS, and this percentage may increase over time.

Q. What is ARC?

A = AIDS

R = Related

C = Complex

ARC is a term that has been widely used by an increasing number of doctors since 1983 to characterise an AIDS-related syndrome that carries a significant but still imprecisely determined likelihood of progression to fully developed AIDS. ARC tends to be marked by two main features:

1) 'Wasting', i.e. an irreversible and rapidly progressive loss of weight;

2) 'Progressive generalised lymphadenopathy' (PGL). This is a generalised swelling and hardening of the lymph nodes/glands which are found in the neck, armpits and groin. The person with ARC may also suffer from skin rashes and diarrhoea.

Q. What is AIDS?

A = Acquired (it's something you get)

I = Immune (resistance to disease)

D = Deficiency (a lack of resistance)

S = Syndrome (a group of signs and symptoms)

A person with AIDS is vulnerable to a number of serious, often fatal 'opportunistic' infections and malignancies. That is, because the body's immune defence system is weakened by HIV infection other ailments can develop without being attacked by these defences. The two most commonly reported opportunistic infections are:

1) A rare form of cancer called 'Kaposi's sarcoma' (KS);

2) A protozoan infection of the lungs known as 'Pneumocystis carini pneumonia' (PCP).

Q. How is the virus passed on?

The virus is very difficult to catch! Because it is an INFECTIOUS and not a CONTAGIOUS disease! Routes of infection include:

1) Sexual contact which involves the exchange of bodily fluids. This is the major route;

2) Infected blood;

3) Infected blood products;

4) Congenitally, i.e. being born from an infected mother. (Also from infected mother's breast milk.)

Q. How widespread is the virus?

TOTAL AIDS CASES

United States	(Mar. 1988)	55,167
Canada	(Feb. 1988)	1,517
New Zealand	(Mar. 1988)	74
Britain	(Feb. 1988)	1,283
Australia	(Feb. 1988)	758
France	(Dec. 1987)	3,073
Germany	(Feb. 1988)	1,848

In the first phase of the epidemic the number of cases has been found to approximately double every six months. After two or three years, this slows down to a doubling time of 10 to 12 months, which is expected to remain fairly constant for several years. This means that a country with 600 cases today will have more than 10,000 cases in four years time, and possibly 100,000 in eight years. In the first years of the epidemic, for each case of AIDS there may be up to 100 or more symptomless but infectious carriers. In the United States, for example, there are thought to be at least 2 million infected people.

REMEMBER: THE VIRUS IS VERY DIFFICULT TO CATCH!

To get ARC or AIDS you have to be infected with HIV. You do NOT get infected with HIV by shaking hands, sharing cutlery, from toilet seats, or from coughs and sneezes. THE DISEASE IS INFECTIOUS BUT NOT CONTAGIOUS!

LIVING WITH U.K. CASES

From 1982, when records were started, up to the time of writing (February 1988), government records show that 720 people had died from the disease out of the known total of 1,283 who have AIDS.

At this date there were 7,007 reported cases of HIV infection. However, the DHSS has indicated that the actual figure of those who are seropositive is more likely to be 30–40,000.

U. K. AIDS CASES TO DATE (February 1988)

Northern	31	(including 22 deaths)
Yorkshire	20	(15)
Trent	22	(8)
East Anglia	18	(12)
NW Thames	572	(284)
NE Thames	239	(141)
SE Thames	115	(69)
SW Thames	45	(28)
Wessex	30	(15)
Oxford	23	(12)
South-Western	22	(18)
West Midlands	21	(16)
Mersey	17	(12)
North-Western	40	(29)
Wales	19	(15)
Scotland	44	(21)
Northern Ireland	5	(3)
Total:	1,283	(720)

The World Health Organisation's figures show that in Britain, with a population of 56 million, the number of cases so far reported represents an incidence of 2.3 per 100,000.

LIVING WITH AFRAIDS

A = Acute

F = Fear

R = Regarding

A = Acquired

I = Immune

D = Deficiency

S = Syndrome

AIDS is frightening! Not to be worried about it, if you are at risk, may be cause for worry in itself.

Reasonable fear or worry may be a sufficient enough spur for a person to accept responsible safer sexual practices.

By contrast, unreasonable fear is likely to lead to anxiety or depression which, in turn, will bring into being a sad, joyless and unsatisfying life.

Unreasonable worry about AIDS can produce 'symptoms' which are similar to AIDS: i.e. loss of weight, sleepless nights, night sweats, loss of energy, etc.

The most effective way to combat unreasonable fear is through education, training and the supply of up to date information.

People who have a reasonable or unreasonable fear of AIDS are often referred to as 'the worried well'. Such people can often be identified by the marked changes in their behaviour. That is, avoiding all contact with anyone suspected of being in a high risk group; constant and unnecessary washing of self, clothes and home; obsessive reading about AIDS; taking the test repeatedly and so on.

Their fear may either be conscious or unconscious. The psychological process called 'denial' may keep away thoughts too troubling for that person to face. It is possible, therefore, for the person to be worrying about AIDS without being aware of it. Give yourself permission to be afraid.

Even when a person actually has HIV his fear of AIDS may still be unreasonable. In my own experience of having HIV, and with the benefit of hindsight, I know that there was a time when my fear was unreasonable.

LIVING WITH CREATIVITY

Being creative is not a minority gift given to the few. Each of us, in our own unique way, has a great reservoir of creative potential. It could well be, for instance, that you or I have the makings of a creative writer, cook, organiser, painter, listener, telephone counsellor, partner or gardener. For most of us, our reservoir of creative potential is largely under-utilised and untapped, and without courageous and repeated explorations will remain that way until the day we die.

Being creative requires repeated effort over time and in various locations. The first time Tchaikovsky addressed the study of music he had within him the potential to write the Swan Lake ballet suite, but the actualisation of it took time, effort, and attentive listening to the tuition of an ever changing reality. That is, he learnt from the influences of his experience of both success and failure during his efforts. However, had he addressed himself to, say, the study of furniture design, he might only have been average. As it was, he found his creative potential, and therefore himself, in the location of music. We may, therefore, have to search in various locations before we find our unique area of creative expanding potential. When we do find it and begin to use it so it will grow in strength. John Lennon had to write some pretty average songs before coming to his classics. It's as though his average writings were needed as foundation stones on which he was then able to build.

I'm not suggesting here that you or I could be a Tchaikovsky or a Lennon. Not least, because the moment I compare myself with another I lose sight of my own uniqueness. I can only be that which I have the potential to become. I can, however, be more fully and creatively myself. The only comparison ever worth making is the one which compares the self I am at this moment with the self I am able to become in the next. None of us are complete. We are each of us perpetually unfinished. Innately in the potential of the next action or moment is the possibility for self-improvement. If I am to face the responsibility for my own improved selfhood then I must allow for the moment of change to be actualised into being. However, I must first want to change, to improve, to push against the boundary of my own creative potential.

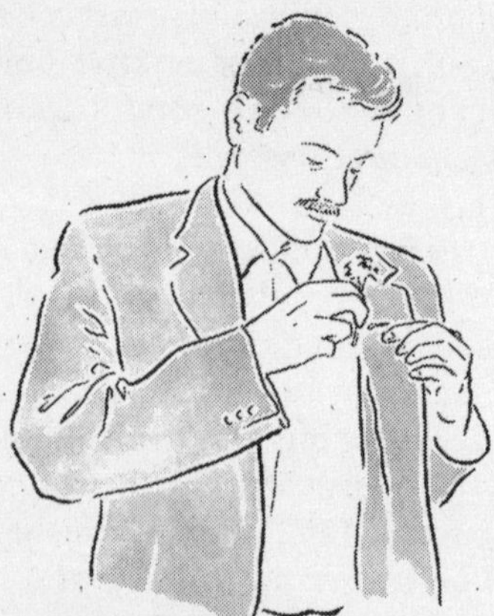

LIVING WITH DARING

Being creative involves us in a kind of daring. It takes courage and daring for any of us to move away from the comparative comfort of our present identity and habits. People may laugh at us as we struggle with our efforts to be creative. They may judge our efforts alongside the creativity of others. They may even condemn the products of our efforts as being unworthy. So what!

Those who know us have a kind of investment in us remaining the same. They don't like us to change, for the moment we do they have to change in relation to us. I recall a boy from my schooldays who was the class comedian. He always had a quick line in humour. Whatever the situation we could rely upon his wit to save the day. When I met him again some years later I barely recognised him. It wasn't that he had changed physically, but he had changed as a person. I had to renegotiate a relationship with him for he was genuinely different. He told me how he had often felt trapped in the role we had cast him in, and it became clear that if I wanted to enjoy his friendship then I must change too. The new person I came to know had always inhabited the old person but had not been recognised by me or my other classmates.

LIVING WITH CHALLENGE

To explore the process of creativity may allow us to utilise our innate potential for it more fully. Joseph Wallas, in his book *The Art of Thought* , states that the creative process consists of four stages: Preparation; Incubation; Illumination and Verification. In stage one the person thinks in a sort of free way, he collects, he searches, listens to suggestions and lets his mind wander. Stage two allows for an internal elaboration and organisation with stage three bringing the solution to the problem. Stage four sees the critical evaluation.

Necessity, it is said, is the mother of invention. If a person is to creatively live with the HIV disease then that person will have to 'invent' a new way of living and being. This will mean the person moving from that which is experienced as being negative to that which is positive. So, let's now examine Wallas' notion of the creative process in relation to having the HIV disease. The following table is not absolute and is offered merely as a rough guide.

POTENTIAL CREATIVE RESPONSES: I		
CREATIVE STAGES	*HIV INFECTION*	*RESPONSES*
One: Preparation	Getting HIV result	Negative
Two: Incubation	Coping with shock, etc.	Negative to positive
Three: Illumination	Facing the challenge	Positive
Four: Verification	Creative adaptation	Positive
THE DESIRED GOAL: SELF-ACTUALISING CREATIVE ACTION		

The time between and at each stage will vary from person to person. In my own case I tend to move from one stage to another, then back again. With each move, however, comes an increased strength of purpose which takes me towards the positive. To move from stage one to stage four took me a full year and still involves me moving backwards and forwards through the stages. Within stage two is a kind of dual experience which I have, more than once, unwittingly allowed myself to construct as being more positive than it actually was or is. The slip from that false position then tends to accentuate the negative. Experience has also taught me that arriving at stage four is no guarantee, in itself, that I am going to stay there. Nonetheless, with increasing courage and daring I constantly aim for the goal of self-actualising creative action.

In his book *The Psychology of the Inventor*, Joseph Rossman used a questionnaire to examine the creative process in some 710 inventors and expanded Wallas' four stages to seven:

1) Observation of a need or difficulty;
2) Analysis of the need;
3) A survey of all available information;
4) A formulation of all objective solutions;
5) A critical analysis of these solutions for their advantages and disadvantages;
6) The birth of a new idea;
7) Experimentation to test out the solution.

As with the previous table, this is again not absolute. It too is no more than a rough guide.

POTENTIAL CREATIVE RESPONSES: II		
STAGE: PROCESS	*HIV DISEASE*	*RESPONSE*
1: Observation	Bad news	Shock
2: Analysis	What now?	Questions
3: Survey	Get the facts	Gathering
4: Formulation	Choices?	Options
5: Analysis	Choose	Selection
6: Birth	Action	Realisation
7: Testing	Deciding	Doing
THE GOAL:	SELF-ACTUALISING CREATIVE ACTIVITY	

LIVING WITH FLOATING EMOTIONS

At each stage in the HIV column of the above table, all seven responses apply and will vary in degree from person to person. That is, when the person is given the bad news that he is HIV infected the initial reaction is likely to be one of shock, coupled with an internal questioning, a surveying of what he knows, a sense of having to make choices from among a range of options, selecting an option in the realisation that it makes sense to him and then carrying out his decision. This process will not be ordered or follow a consistent pattern. It is much more likely that the person will experience an emotional floating of the kind which shifts him from clear logical and conscious thought through to unclear unconscious reactions and back again. Though apparently in control of himself, he is likely to be confused and should be given the time, within that confused state, to express himself however he chooses. He may very well say and do things which he later regrets. He should be reassured that his behaviour is perfectly normal under the circumstances. He should be allowed to experience the negatives in his own way for these are the very building blocks on which he may later build a positive life.

LIVING WITH ACTION

In both of the creative processes so far discussed we can see that each begins with doing something. In the first table we see that 'preparation' is the start, while in the second 'observation' begins the process. Creativity does not, therefore, evolve by pure spontaneous generation. Rather, it evolves or emerges out of action. It is only through the action involved in creatively exploring a wide range of options and locations that intuition can find the right soil to grow in. The quick and ready insight we gain from intuition has its roots firmly established in courageous searching. In other words, we get out what we put in.

This 'stages approach' in explaining and understanding the creative process is also explored by A. F. Osborn in the book *Applied Imagination* and by M. I. Stein in two books: *Creativity and Culture* and *Stimulating Creativity*. However, W. E. Vinacke, in *The Psychology of Thinking* was highly critical of the notion of stages, pointing out that some creative work is worked and reworked, then reworked again through time. (This I know from experience to be true in my case.) Nonetheless, both contributions are useful here. I tend to the view that there is an element of truth in both and that neither is absolute. Our eclecticism here should allow us to take and use those elements which enhance our unique grasp of the creative process.

LIVING WITH FREUD

Freud offers, as an explanation of creativity, unconscious motivations and sublimations which, he claims, are attempts to solve conflicts. That is, the person is unable to actualise his instinctive sexuality or aggression and unconsciously finds other ways to express the potency of them through creativity. In Dr Humberto Nagera's study of Van Gogh the author claims that the energy required for his paintings was nothing less than modified sexual energy. The notion here is 'the more sexual activity, the less art', which does not hold up to close inspection. As Anthony Storr points out in his book *The Dynamics of Creation*, 'Quite a number of creative people have led rather active sexual lives without apparently diminishing their artistic production.' I cannot go along with Freud at all on this. Not least because of his notion that the creative person is not far removed from neurosis. What utter rot! The simple truth, if we are to accept the notion of neurosis at all, is that none of us are far from neurosis. It is part of what it means to be human.

LIVING WITH DESTRUCTION

What, then, is creativity? In simple terms it is the ability to bring something new into being. However, it is more than that, it is a chosen act which enables the emergence and development of something unique for the specific individual. Thus, creation exists in potential long before it is actualised. More than that, creation innately takes into account both the potential and the limitations of the creator. That is, I can only create that which I have the potential to create. Nonetheless, it is only through pushing against the flexible boundary of my potential that I can explore and perhaps discover latent possibilities. When worked upon, perhaps more than once, this may increase the range of my potential and thereby decrease my limitations. I can only find out by doing. In 'doing' I increase my involvement in the positive recreation of my-self. I am what I do. I do not, however, always do what I am capable of becoming. The challenge I face here is, who do I elect to become? And, which parts of my negative destructivity do I allow to die off or be killed off, through an act of will, so that I might increase my creativity?

When I allow those negative and destructive aspects of my-self to die off or be killed off, by an act of will, I do so not to rid myself of them through some psychological act of denial, but through the conscious act of choosing. In so doing I facilitate their decaying nature being transformed or converted into a creative fertilising agent, into which I may safely and with assurance plant my seeds of creativity.

I am creative only when I choose to be. The constant rebirthing of my positive creativity, if it is to be actualised, must therefore involve the constant process of my negative destructivity dying. Thus there can be no creativity without some degree of prior destruction and, paradoxically, there can be no destruction without some degree of creation resulting. Which came first is a chicken-and-egg kind of argument, the pursuit of which will keep us, in human terms, merely statically and permanently facing the blank screen of ignorant wonder. Onto this screen we may then publicly display the bliss of our unknowing fanciful projections. That is, we have not the slightest idea about the particular phenomenon, and instead of saying so we continuously speculate in a manner which deludes us into thinking we understand it. Furthermore, we try our best to convince the other viewers of our 'understanding' of the 'truth'. The question of which is the stronger or more potent may lead us to the same blank screen if we do not take into account the interrelatedness and interdependence of and between creation and destruction. To grapple with this notion unaided is unreasonable. If I am to understand it better I am required firstly to grasp the notion that every action produces another. In human terms, this means that the only consistent factor of be-ing is change.

LIVING WITH FREEDOM

Everything I do will have some degree of impact on those with whom I relate, and what they then do in response will have an impact upon me, and so on. This is the human dynamic. The challenge I face here is that I am free to act and, to a large extent, react, either through the process of conscious choice or otherwise. I will always have to react, so why not be more in control of how I opt to do so?

What then when the dynamic is a combination of human and human infection? Specifically, what when the human is affected by the actions of the HIV disease? In simple terms the disease will, to some degree or another, react to me according to how I react to it, and I will react to the disease according to how it reacts within me. Let me give you an example of this: When I was told that I had the HIV disease (the action) my initial response and felt experience (the reaction) was largely one of spontaneous, instant and shocking emotional pain. I felt dirty, guilty and ashamed. The sense of dirt was compounded by the realisation that I could not be cleansed of it. The guilt emerged out of my unwanted Catholic upbringing about the 'sins of homosexuality'. Despite the fact that I'd been out for many years, the shame was in part about being found out. More than that, however, it was also about the way I was reacting. These reactions were not thought through logically at the time. They were fleeting and floating emotions and as such were a reflection of the unwanted baggage I'd carried around with me for years. How I loathed owning those reactions. My HIV disease had, at that time, the perfect host in which to do its worst. Where had all my development gone?

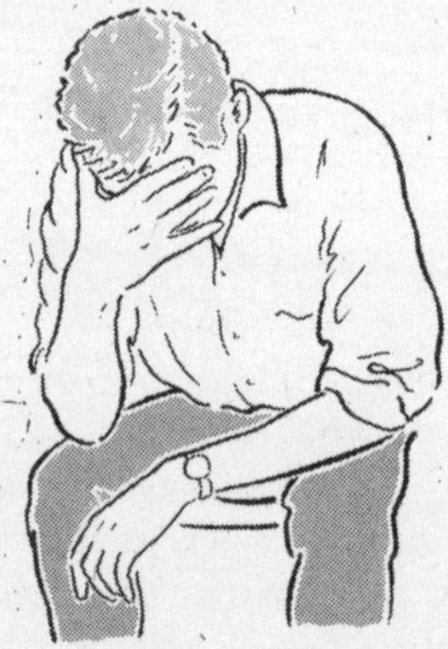

LIVING WITH ANXIOUS DEPRESSION

What I was then unaware of was that at the centre of these reactions was an anger turned inwards towards self. I wish I could have known that at the time, for the result was severe depression. This depression was difficult both for others and for myself to recognise because I was then unwilling to acknowledge its existence. So unprepared and unwilling was I to actually consciously own the depression that I effectively disguised it behind a convincing mask of coping. However, lurking within its depths was an urge to negatively self-destruct. I hated these weak-willed thoughts and therefore myself for having them. This in turn fuelled the negative self-concept and flow of anger inwards towards the very centre of my being. The question 'Why me?' was answered inside by my own inner judgemental 'Because you deserve it, the way you've lived!'

In this negative state I tended to view only the negative side of everything else, especially when there was a possible ambiguity. Take the following lines which in reality are about a man's grief at the death of his daughter and see if you can see how they became twisted to suit my dispiritedness:

> Had you restrained your love, you would be free of sorrow. The greater the love, while one possesses it, the greater the sorrow when one is deprived of it ... unpleasure must follow pleasure...
>
> Von Tepl (c. 1400)

LIVING WITH REACTIONS

I'll come back, a little later, to the feeling associated with first receiving the results of my HIV test. Before doing so, however, there is the flip side of reacting to take into account. That is, pro-acting. When I simply react, as I did, there is a kind of inner message which says, 'I am a victim of something over which I have absolutely no control and I can do nothing about it.' In contrast to this, my pro-active inner message says, 'I can and I will do something about this.' There is no such person as the completely re- or pro-active person. We all exist somewhere between the two. However, we can with increased insight move more towards pro-activity and with effort and courage remain there for increasingly longer periods. Nonetheless, we should not lose sight of the fact that there are times when it right to react. Indeed, not to react under certain circumstances would be quite impossible. The point is, however, that we don't have to remain in that condition for ever. Not only are we capable of becoming more pro-active but it is also beneficial to our health to become so.

RE-ACTIVE	PRO-ACTIVE	I AM	CHANGES TO MAKE
Conforming	Disobedient		
Victim	Activist		
Helpless	Resourceful		
Follower	Leader		
Inactive	Active		
Consumer	Producer		
Abuser	User		
Depressed	Angry		
Static	Changing		
Selfish	Selfful		
Accepts	Initiates		
Expects	Gives		

In the re-active and pro-active table there are no right or wrong places to be. We have to face up to where we are and what we intend to do about it. The challenge I face here is to move through negative experiences into more positive ones. To do that here will involve me in being more open with you. Being more open is like making oneself more visible so that more of oneself may be seen.

LIVING WITH ISOLATION

When a person is given the news that he has the HIV disease he is quite free to share that news with whoever he chooses. Equally, he is free to keep the news to himself. However, should he choose the latter course he is in danger of further isolating himself, which may indicate that he is not in control of his environment or himself. Such a person may feel that he is justified in keeping the news to himself for all kinds of reasons, not least the possible loss of a job. Nonetheless, he is free to select whom he tells. If he feels that there is absolutely no one with whom he can share the news then the chances are that he is already isolated and in need of considerable support. Being in control of one's environment and oneself means that the person does not wait for life to happen to him. Rather, he pro-actively creates the happening and dictates the direction of his life.

LIVING VISIBLY

The challenge I face here is to be that much more open with you. To be more visible. To do that will involve me in being more subjective than I have thus far been. I must invite you into a close encounter with my feelings at and shortly after the time I discovered I had the HIV disease. After I was given the diagnosis I kept a diary as a means of helping myself to explore my feelings. Some months later, I reflected on what I had written and made further notes. What follows, then, are a couple of diary entries and the reflections subsequently made. These are the feelings and thoughts of an incomplete human being at a time of major crisis. However, thanks largely to the crisis itself I have changed a great deal, as has my lifestyle and environment:

> ...It was Friday 11th July 1986 at half past one in the afternoon when I found out that I had the virus...
>
> Despite my awareness of the possibilities I was not in the least prepared for the news. Though outwardly calm I went instantly into shock. I recall the doctor gently telling me through a dark cloud that I also had a severe case of herpes, a fungal infection and pneumonia and that I should have to be admitted on the spot. I had great difficulty following what he was saying for each word he spoke became immediately transformed into that word, DEATH. I was aware of the duality of what he was saying and of what echoed within. Confusion rebounded in my head till it hurt and I wanted to run like hell. This wasn't happening to me. I don't want it. I damn well refuse to own this disease. There must be some mistake. I heard myself refuse point blank to be admitted. Was he not, after all, telling me to come in to die? How dare he! The more gently insistent he became the more aggressively defensive I heard myself responding. I was shocked at my own behaviour. Another doctor was brought and I was given a complete physical examination. The doctor's touch gave me great comfort. Eventually, I was allowed home with massive doses of antibiotics and on the understanding that I would return at the slightest sign of the pneumonia getting worse. I remained in that deep shock for the remainder of the day, taking

taxis from one cafe to another, leaving £5 tips wherever I went. It proved to be a most expensive day.

All the ills passed as the antibiotics did their work over the next couple of weeks, but for some time afterwards I became increasingly preoccupied with thoughts of death. I so wanted to talk about death in general and of my death in particular but people, otherwise kind, caring people, refused to allow me. An irritating pattern began to emerge. I would talk about the very real possibility of going on to develop 'full-blown AIDS' and of the known outcome, death. My friends, not hearing the meaning behind what I was saying, would invariably counter with, 'Well you could get knocked down in the road tomorrow...' or, 'Death comes to us all at some time...' I knew that they were trying to comfort me but they were not dealing with it or me very effectively and their comments left me feeling angry. They too wanted to run like hell and make believe that it wasn't true. I had to fight to get them to listen to what concerned me. With many, I gave up quite quickly as an act of compassion, for they suffered in attempting to talk about my possible death. Besides, we didn't have a shared language to help us get through to the heart of the meaning.

I would much prefer the comfort of religious faith but I have none. Not even to blame. I am utterly alone...

In an attempt to find someone to talk to about my state of shock, my illness and possible death I telephoned a well-known psychotherapy centre, one to which I was known and had been a client of. They refused to even see me. I was frankly amazed but felt the positive potential of my anger rise once again within me at this rejection. The fighting spirit was at least alive and well. Courage was becoming more important by the day.

Courage, however, was not always available when it was needed. I found myself becoming depressed and more than once thoughts of suicide — a chance to decide — came to me. Thoughts I was ashamed of and felt I couldn't ever share with others. Not least, because I constantly reminded myself that had I not been gay then this would never have happened to me. Perhaps those Jesus freaks were right and this was the result of a wasted life. Thoughts like these, and others far more extreme, came and went. I was becoming scared of cracking up completely. I came to know that the growing depression was anger turned inwards towards self, but despite the intellectual awareness I was then unable to do much about it. I began to hate myself and everything gay.

At the point of an all-time low I telephoned someone I'd met through a friend. A man who was well versed in the issues of the HIV disease. Within minutes of speaking to T. W. I found myself crying. I'd never cried like this. My whole body was involved. I hurt all over. T. W. came to my home and the first thing he said was, 'I've no intention of counselling you.' Instead he put his arms around me and stroked me. I burst into tears and cried and shouted for hours on end. He never once let go. Here was a man who knew the language needed to get to the meaning. I attempted to move away from time to time but he saw the meaning and held me even more gently. How lucky I was to know such a man. Afterwards, we talked. He gave me space to talk through all my crazy and not so crazy thoughts. All the anger and pain came flooding out and so too did the depression. It has not troubled me since. When he left, hours later, I felt safe with myself.

I telephoned H. D. S. to tell her how I was feeling like a leper and how I'd been thinking of getting myself a bell to ring. She listened. When I stopped, she offered me advice on the kind of bell I might consider suitable. She discounted church bells, me being a humanist and them being too heavy, and settled on a bicycle bell. Within minutes she had me laughing. It was a good feeling. Through the humour I could see how crazy my thoughts were. She laughed with me and I knew instinctively that she wasn't laughing at me. Sure my thoughts were kind of crazy but they were also quite funny too.

I watched an American television production with my dearest and closest friend B. K. who had just arrived back from a holiday abroad. It was called *Buddies* and was about a young man dying of AIDS and the other young man who came to befriend him and act as his 'buddy'. Anyway, there was a scene when the buddy asks the AIDS patient what he would do if he had just one healthy day. I found myself getting into quite a state as my mind played with the notion. I guess what I was feeling was a kind of grief, for my mind played the same scene over and over again. I was kissing and hugging all my nephews and nieces.

Despite the great need I have to be held and loved I still feel scared when someone hugs me or kisses my face. The bottom line is that I don't want to contaminate them. I still often feel dirty and to blame. Intellectually I have enough knowledge to realise that there is absolutely no reason in the world to stop kissing just as I realise that I am not to blame for having the virus. But my emotions twist and distort the logical and rational into a shape which reflects the virus itself. When I pull back from a hug or a kiss it is myself I'm pulling away from, not you. T. W. understood that very well.

I'm capable of becoming almost completely paranoid at the slightest sign of infection in others. I don't mean those with the virus. I mean those with the common cold, those with a slight cough and those with throat infections. I'm so aware that my immune defence system is at risk and that I may not be able to physically deal with the next sneeze. I sometimes just want to shut myself away from everyone and from time to time that's just what I do. When I've done so without real justification, however, I've become so lonely that I now try, often with great effort, to keep up social contacts.

After the diagnosis and for many months afterwards I lost all interest in sex. I had, in effect, switched off. Since that time (and up to the time of this diary entry) I have not had sex with another person. My doctor and friends often speak about safer sex and of how I should explore the possibilities. For reasons much to do with the fear of contaminating others who do not have the virus and of being contaminated by others who may have other sexually transmittable diseases I cannot bring myself to have sex with another person. Learning once again, however, through masturbation, to explore, value and enjoy my sexual nature and my-self has been difficult but has proved a powerful and worthwhile experience. Creating fantasy images within and for myself was helped by erotic poetry, novels and borrowed videos. Nonetheless, my level of sexual activity has decreased considerably from what it once was. I grieve the loss often.

Within those diary entries and subsequent reflections are thoughts and ideas of which I am now both variously proud, slightly ashamed of, and a little embarrassed both to admit to and to have actually had. That was a time, however, of major crisis in my life and I need to remind myself that it is okay for me to have had such thoughts and ideas. It's not thoughts and ideas which define me, it is what I do NOW that matters. Those same thoughts and ideas, like John Lennon's early songs, can with effort, courage and application be the very foundation stones which I can and do intend to build upon. Indeed, I would go so far as to say that without that crisis in my life I would not now be growing at the rate I am. Giving the crisis freedom to express itself has allowed me to reap huge rewards.

LIVING POSITIVELY

If I am to continue to grow through this disease, if I am to unload unwanted baggage, if I am to emerge a better person because of it and not despite it, if I am to focus on the quality and not the quantity of my existence, if I am not to remain humanly static, if I am to be realistic about my condition, if I am to be courageous, then I must take up the challenge to find the creative potential of the disease. There are a lot of 'ifs' in those statements, so the first thing I must do is to unload them. Let me offer those same statements but this time without the 'ifs' and without the negatives.

BEING POSITIVE

1. I will grow through this infection;
2. I will unload unwanted baggage;
3. I will emerge a better person because of it;
4. I will focus on the quality of my life;
5. I will become more humanly mobile;
6. I will defeat permanent reactive depression;
7. I will be realistic about my condition;
8. I will be courageous;
9. I will search for the creative elements;
10. I will take up the challenge.

LIVING WITHIN REASON

The challenge here is to unashamedly remind myself that those ten goals are not some kind of magic formula but are all perfectly reasonable, realistic and attainable goals well within my human potential to achieve.

Alternatively (there are always alternatives) I may, through the negative reaction of allowing myself to be nothing more than a consumer of my HIV disease, become emotionally, psychologically, socially and spiritually invalided to it. I could become hooked on the genuine sympathy and caring of others and adopt a passive consumer role. To do so, however, would entail me becoming part of my own compost out of which the only thing to grow would be the caring of others. Damn it, I won't go that way. The challenge here is to be positive and I damn well will be.

I WILL

1. I will care for myself;
2. I will take charge of my life;
3. I will accept responsibility for my life;
4. I will be a producer not a consumer;
5. I will acknowledge my potential;

6. I will

7. I will

8. I will

9. I will

10. I will

LIVING WITH OPEN-MINDED CARING

By far the most important issue in being positive is that of caring. Preparing the way for open-minded caring is not an easy task, for most of us carry within ourselves a kind of confused understanding of what it is to care.

Before I am able to address the notion of caring, however, I must first open my mind to the possibilities. That is, I must clear my mind of blockages and obstacles. To do that, I must remind myself what a closed mind is.

> A closed mind is one which has a relatively high degree of isolation, contradiction and accentuation of belief-disbelief difference, and which is poorly differentiated, especially in its disbelief subsystem. The system tends to be frozen, static, resistant to change and intolerant of ambiguity and uncertainty; the individual knows what is true and what is false, what is right and what is wrong, and has no intention of altering his views. People with closed minds tend to interpret experience as always confirming what they already know.

What then, is an open mind? The same writer goes on to say:

> The open mind is by contrast a growing and developing system; it is so to speak perpetually unfinished. Not only is there a continuing and spontaneous tendency for the elements within it to be brought into new relationships with each other and thereby modified, but the system as a

> whole is sensitively responsive to the tuition of a changing reality.
>
> Derek Wright (1971)

I recognise myself only too clearly in Derek Wright's notion of the closed mind, but I also recognise my potential in his notion of the open mind. For me to achieve this open mind means that I must step from that which I know and feel comfortable with into the relatively unexplored areas of self. The challenge here is to do so with courage. When I act in courage I acknowledge the greater mystery of selfhood whilst more fully being able to recognise the universe outside of my own existence. I become the evolving creator of the person I call self and I come to realise that I and I alone am responsible for the directions my life takes. To look back or attempt, through whatever mechanism, to go back, is to sink beneath the existence of the present and future potential.

Victor Frankl, in his remarkable book *Man's Search for Meaning*, writes about his time in a German concentration camp, and tells of those who let themselves decline because they could not see a future goal. Such people find themselves occupied with retrospective thoughts.

> They preferred to close their eyes and to live in the past. Life for such people became meaningless...
>
> V. Frankl (1971)

LIVING IN THE 'NOW'

We too are free to close our eyes and our minds and live in the past, but what meaning does that have in the now? I am not defined by what I did but by what I do NOW. I must be willing to let go of those things which have already gone if I am to achieve an identity and meaning in the present. The challenge here is to find meanings. In my efforts, I open myself to the freedom to choose in the now and it blows my mind. I discover that it is I, that it has been I, who chooses who I am now and who I am to become in the future. To be free to embrace more fully the art of be-ing myself in the next moment I must accept responsibility for the existence which is me. Above all else I must learn to love myself. To step into the unexplored area of self is to step into the potentiality of selfhood and that requires that I do so with love. That love will give me the courage to face that which I will meet — myself.

LIVING WITH LOVE

> To love is a productive activity. It implies caring for, knowing, responding, affirming, enjoying: the person, the tree, the painting, the idea. It means bringing to life, increasing his/her aliveness. It is a process, self-renewing and self-increasing.
>
> E. Fromm (1978)

I have to work hard at loving self. I seem more capable of loving others. It's as though the love I have, the love which in my heart I know I am, must leave my very body and be transmitted outwards for it to be love. The challenge I face here is to allow that same love to be generated inwards in such a way that I don't feel selfish. However, the knowledge I have of my failings and weaknesses tends to block the way, as does the social script which says, 'To love self is selfish'. The assumption being that to the degree that I love myself I cannot love others. This notion goes back a long way. Both Calvin and Freud played a part in generating it. Calvin, by calling self-love a 'pest', and Freud, by assuming that self-love was the libido turned inwards towards self and therefore a kind of narcissism. The challenge I face here is to remind myself that the affirmation of my own life, happiness, growth and freedom is rooted in my capacity to love with care, respect, responsibility and knowledge. If I am to love productively, then I must love myself too. If I can only love others then I cannot really love at all. You will recall how I said earlier that in being positive the most important aspect to consider was that of caring. This is another way of saying, loving. However, the term 'caring' has become a cliche through overuse and inappropriate use. The English phrase 'Take care of yourself' is fast becoming as meaningless as the American 'Have a nice day'. Nonetheless, taking care of myself is the challenge I face here.

LIVING WITH CARING

Caring is NOT just a matter of good intentions and warm regard. Caring demands an activity, an involvement, a taking into account. In his little yet huge book *On Caring*, Milton Mayeroff tells us that the major ingredients of caring are Knowing; Alternating Rhythms; Patience; Honesty; Trust; Humility; Hope and Courage. It may help to link 'self' where the word 'other' is used.

KNOWING

> To care for someone, I must know many things. I must know, for example, who the other is, what his powers and limitations are, what his needs are, and what is conducive to his growth; I must know how to respond to his needs, and what my own powers and limitations are.

ALTERNATING RHYTHMS

> I cannot care by sheer habit; I must be able to learn from my past. I see what my actions amount to, whether I have helped or not, and, in the light of the results, maintain or modify my behaviour so that I can better help the other.

PATIENCE

> Patience is not waiting passively for something to happen, but is a kind of participation with the other in which we give fully of ourselves. And it is misleading to understand patience simply in terms of time, for we give the other space as well. By patiently listening to the distraught

man, by being present for him, we give him space to think and feel.

HONESTY

Honesty is present in caring as something positive, and not as a matter of not doing something, not telling lies or not deliberately deceiving others. This meaning of honesty may be suggested by the phrase 'to be honest with oneself', where this includes actively confronting and being open to oneself. In caring I am honest in trying to see truly. To care for the other, I must see the other as it is and not as I would like it to be or feel it must be.

TRUST

Trusting the other is to let go; it includes an element of risk and a leap into the unknown, both of which take courage.

HUMILITY

The man who cares is generally humble in being ready and willing to learn more about the other and himself...the problem is one of appropriateness to this novel situation, and this situation is, generally speaking, not simply a repetition of the past requiring only a mechanical application of principles.

HOPE

Such hope is not an expression of the insufficiency of the present in comparison with the sufficiency of a hoped-for future; it is rather an expression of the plenitude of the present, a present alive with a sense of the possible.

COURAGE

> Trust in the other to grow and in my own ability to care gives me courage to go into the unknown, but it is also true that without the courage to go into the unknown such trust would be impossible. And clearly, the greater the sense of going into the unknown, the more courage is called for in caring.
>
> M. Mayeroff (1971)

When I care for myself I give myself the opportunity to explore my needs and my potential; I give myself room to grow into; I learn and change; I listen to every aspect of my human functioning; I think and explore my feelings; I search after truth; I face reality; I let go of that which must be let go; I see the unknown as being full of potential; I adapt; I grasp the present opportunities with courage and celebrate my uniqueness. When I do all of this I also love.

When I care for myself as a man living with HIV disease I must go even further. That is, I must become more finely attuned to each of the aspects listed above and I must examine closely each element of my human functioning to see which areas need strengthening. But what is meant here by 'human functioning'?

We function in four areas, that is, physically, psychologically, socially and culturally, and spiritually. When our functioning is balanced there is a kind of harmony in and between each area. However, when there is discord or disease in just one of these areas all the other areas are to some extent affected.

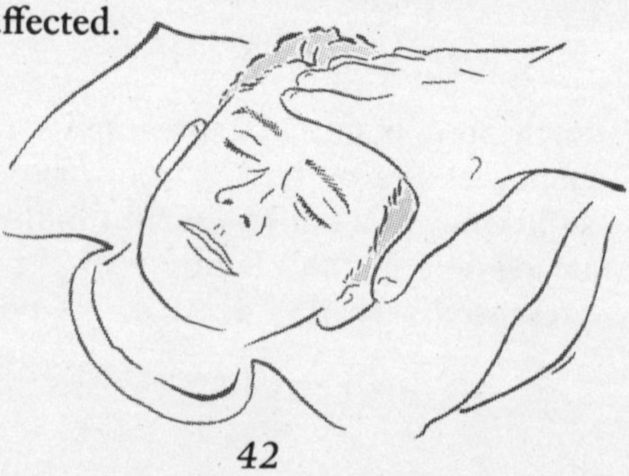

LIVING WITH THE FULL SELF

As a person with HIV disease I am not just affected physically, even though the disease is primarily physical in nature. All the other areas of my functioning are affected also. You will recall from my diary entries just how much, at that time of major crisis, my psychological functioning came under attack. It is as though the weakening of one area sets off a weakening reaction in the other areas. Taking care of my-self, therefore, must involve me in taking care in and of all four areas:

PHYSICAL FUNCTIONING: Growth, development and maintenance of the body. *This includes being sexual.*

PSYCHOLOGICAL FUNCTIONING: Mental, intellectual, thinking, fantasy. *This includes being sexual.*

SOCIAL AND CULTURAL FUNCTIONING: Interpersonal and social relationships, creative awareness, expression and appreciation. *This includes being sexual.*

SPIRITUAL FUNCTIONING: The animating or vital force of living. This does not exclude those of us who are either atheist or agnostic. *This includes being sexual.*

LIVING WITH SEXUALITY

It won't have escaped your notice in the previous section that each heading has an emphasised sentence 'This includes being sexual.' There are good reasons for this. Not least to emphasise that being sexual is only in one part being genital. Even when a person stops giving any physical expression to his sexual nature he does not stop being sexual. A more accurate description, therefore, of the celibate would be the sexual-celibate. Another reason for the underlined statement is to show that the notion of 'safer sex' is not restricted to the physical acts of being sexual. Responsible safer sex takes account of all four areas. Indeed, safer sex must include all the elements listed earlier under caring and loving. When people speak of safer sex in purely physical terms what they actually mean, or what is in danger of being understood, is safer genitality. Because of this, and because of the confusion inherent in the term safer sex, I much prefer the term 'safer sexuality'.

LIVING WITH CRISIS

Whether I am to care for others with the HIV disease or myself as a person with it will, at some stage or another, involve me, either directly or indirectly, in a crisis, or crisis situations. People usually ask for help when they have 'a problem', 'a need', when they are 'under stress' or are 'in crisis'. These familiar terms are often used interchangeably and to such an extent that we tend to attribute, or are in danger of attributing, the same meaning to each term. Yet how we, as individuals or agencies, conceptualise the state of being will largely affect the response, the manner of the response, the structure and ethos of an agency, the techniques employed and the deployment of resources.

When I was first given my diagnosis and for some time afterwards, I entered into and remained in a state of crisis for many months. I was also under stress. That is, one of my responses to the crisis state was stress. A state of crisis is not an illness but stress does have pathogenic potential. Stress is a kind of burden under which I could crack up. By contrast, however, crisis has an inherent growth-promoting potential. The social theorist W. I. Thomas saw crisis as a catalyst that disturbs old habits, evokes new responses, and becomes a major factor in charting new development. Looked at in that way, a crisis is a call to new action. The challenge it provokes in many who live with HIV disease, for example, helps them create new coping mechanisms which serve in turn to strengthen their adapting ability and improve their mental health.

As a person striving to maintain a state of equilibrium throughout my HIV disease, by a whole range of adaptive changes, I also went through various stages of perception about my HIV infection during the crisis. I should point out, however, that periods of crisis don't actually have a neat and identifiable beginning, a middle and an end. The various stages tend to flow into, between and around each other where they are compounded.

THE CRISIS		
STAGES & HOW VIEWED THROUGH TIME		*RESULT*
First:	As a threat to integrity	Anxiety
Second:	As loss and deprivation	Depression
Third:	As a challenge	Energy

Arriving at stage three took me quite some time because of my unwillingness to accept and deal with the diagnosis creatively.

LIVING WITH A SECOND CHANCE

Throughout the various stages listed in the table above, old problems long since dealt with began to surface in my mind. In so doing I was, paradoxically, given a kind of 'second chance' to deal with them again, and this time more effectively.

The period of crisis will vary from person to person and will eventually come to an end. Before it does, however, one of three internal processes is likely to occur:

1. The HIV diagnosis will be accepted by the person;
2. The HIV diagnosis will be blamed on someone else;
3. The HIV diagnosis will be rejected by the person.

LIVING WITH HIV

The person who does not resolve the crisis in one of the ways listed in the previous section is likely to enter a state of unresolved mental disorganisation. You will recall from my diary entries that I initially rejected the diagnosis. That is, I couldn't bring myself to accept it and I also looked for someone or something to blame it on. This rejection was little more than an internal attempt to resolve the crisis. The attempt, of course, failed and I eventually had to accept that I was infected. The person who, by whatever mechanism, opts for number one of the three is more likely to make creative readjustments and form rewarding inner and outer relationships.

A useful helping mechanism for us all to be aware of is that a person in crisis is highly susceptible to the influence of significant others. In my case it was a man who refused to counsel me and held me instead. The helping person should aim to do as little as possible for the person in crisis.

The little, well thought through, well directed and well timed is far more effective than too much intervention.

Even when the crisis is over it is still likely that the person will be experiencing some degree of grief. The degrees of this will vary both within and between different people. Such grief will also be experienced by the partner/s, friends and family of the person infected, especially when it is obvious that the person is going to or is about to die. Or, indeed, when it is feared that death will result.

LIVING WITH EXILES

In living memory there is little to compare the grief impact of HIV disease with. We could look to natural disasters for a comparison but they have more of a community, national or internationally based impact. Individual soldiers fighting a war, the making of which they had little or nothing whatsoever to do with, comes closest. They are a 'high risk' group of individuals collectively seen as one. When one dies the grief is experienced first individually and then, hopefully, collectively.

As with all wars, the war being waged against HIV disease will have no 'winners' in the sense of an outright victory. The only victors are those who will come through it with an enhanced humanity. In every war the power behind the propaganda machine actively encourages man to hate man, for it then becomes easier to kill your enemy.

In the war against HIV disease there are those who choose to alienate themselves from the fight. In so doing, they then have to rationalise their separation from those affected by hating them. 'It's not my war, I want no part of it, it's their own fault for getting involved in the first place...' In their opting out these righteous exiles alienate themselves from their own humanity and become less than human. I grieve for them.

LIVING WITH GRIEF

The enormous increase in grief related to HIV disease over the last seven years suggests that an enhanced understanding of its nature be considered by us all. An experience of grief is likely to begin at the acute end of the scale, then, with its working through, move to a less acute stage. A person recently given the diagnosis of HIV disease may misinterpret their natural grief reactions and confuse these with the signs and symptoms of the disease itself. A person experiencing grief is likely to have a marked tendency to sighing, which may be thought of as a breathing problem. He is likely to experience a loss of strength and a sense of exhaustion, which may be thought of as being more to do with the disease. It is likely, also, that the person will have either a reduced or an increased appetite. During my own period of crisis I put on over two and a half stones in weight.

LIVING WITH DISTORTED VIEWS

In crisis and grief our perceptions are likely to become distorted. It would be highly unreasonable to expect a person in crisis to maintain a clear view of things throughout the crisis. We are likely to say and do things which don't make sense either to others or to ourselves. The HIV test results crisis is little understood but one example was reported in the press: When the man was given his positive result his internal reaction was to wish for 'full-blown AIDS' to develop so he could get the whole thing over with. His views changed after the crisis had run its course.

Whenever a person is given a positive result it might, therefore, be wise for the doctor to ask the patient to suspend acting on any internal response for a period of at least six weeks.

SOME DISTORTED REACTIONS	ME, YES or NO?	YOU, YES or NO?
Overactivity without a sense of loss	no	
An acquisition of other symptoms	yes, at first and in part	
Psychosomatic conditions develop	yes, though not major	
Alterations in relationships	yes, locking myself away	
Furious hostility towards specific others	yes, at my doctor	
Emotional woodenness	no	
Loss of initiating behaviour	yes, for a while	
Social or economic abandonment	yes, gave £5 tips in cafes	
Agitated depression	yes	

There are no 'proper' or 'right' reactions to crisis or grief. There are only the ones we have. Those who are prepared, through talking and experiencing consciously, to do the 'crisis work' and 'grief work' at an early stage, however, are much more likely to heal quicker. Whilst this 'working through' cannot and should not be forced, it can nonetheless be enabled or facilitated by sensitive, well-timed and minimal intervention.

LIVING WITH CREATIVE INTERVENTION

Creative intervention is more an art than a science and will take into account that a person with HIV disease is not a problem to be solved but a mystery to be apprehended.

In the presence of that mystery the caring person, like the good doctor, does as little as possible.

Nor is the person with the disease there for us to experience our caring through. Without that person to care for what would we do with our caring?

The kind of caring which makes the experience of caring more important than the action is selfishness.

True caring needs not an ounce of practice for it comes through do-ing and be-ing.

To care productively is to abandon self to the point where the self is second and thus becomes more full. Such caring is selfless. Such caring seeks no rewards.

LIVING THROUGH BE-ING

There are no easy methods of dealing with HIV disease. Nonetheless, there are things we can do to foster the right conditions so that we may then be more able to creatively deal with ourselves. We can start by:

BE-ING ALONE: Be-ing alone is not the same as loneliness for the person is in the company of himself. Be-ing alone allows us to get away from external stimulations and listen to ourselves more fully. Listen to the sounds and resources of your own potential. Let it echo freely within. Listen and become more attuned. Offer no resistance. Listen to who you are and who you can become. Be-ing alone means that we must be disobedient to the gregarious demands to always be in the company of others. Be-ing with others too much means that we miss out on be-ing with ourselves.

BE-ING INACTIVE: People with HIV disease who strive to be creative should, whenever possible, give themselves long periods of time for thinking and feeling. They should disobey the demands of routine, for routine stifles the creative process. Be-ing inactive is to take time off to 'do' nothing. It is not about withdrawing or being lazy. Be-ing inactive allows us to create a safe space in which to creatively explore our inner potential.

BE-ING A DAYDREAMER: Daydreaming is a wonderful resource. It allows us to enter a fantasy life which has the innate potential of opening up whole new realms of growth and discovery.

BE-ING A FREE THINKER: Be-ing a free thinker implies that the person unashamedly allows his thoughts to wander without judgement or restraint in whatever direction the thoughts move in. This is not the same as analytical free association. For there is a demand there to offer up, through the spoken word, and that means some kind of prior organisation before speaking.

BE-ING A FISHERMAN OF IDEAS: When we allow the mind to wander we should attempt to go with it and be ready to fish out those creative linking thoughts which lead from one idea to the next. Especially when there are linking similarities. This is a major source of what it means to be creative.

BE-ING OPEN: Be-ing open means being able to suspend all judgements and criticisms for a period of time. It means a willingness to explore in a kind of naive innocent sort of way before rejecting anything.

BE-ING AN ACTION-REPLAYER: It is often assumed that once a person has moved through a crisis or trauma then it is best to forget it. Such 'forgetting' may, however, require great efforts of mental suppression. Suffering in silence is too highly valued in our culture. To replay old conflicts, traumas and crises will give us the opportunity to more effectively deal with them. We can do this alone or with a soul friend.

BE-ING A RESOLVER: Working through new and old conflicts in a creative way allows us to explore alternative resolutions. When I find the courage and create for myself the opportunity to do so, like in the writing on this page, the inherent conflicts of the content, and within myself, are given resolved meanings.

BE-ING ALERT: Be-ing alert allows us to recognise either suddenly, gradually, or through time those links and ideas which we had previously dismissed as insignificant, accidental or inconsequential. Be-ing alert allows us to see the area where previously there was insufficient awareness.

LIVING WITH A CENTRE

Be-ing sick and be-coming better is the major challenge I face. By becoming better I do not mean being cured. I mean exactly what I say, becoming better. I spoke earlier about being depressed and being anxious in a way which may have misled you. Let me clear that up now. Being anxious is not something which happens to me, it is something I become and, therefore, when it occurs, it is something I am. When anxiety is evoked within me I am anxious. Anxiety is not something I have but is something I am. I am, therefore, everything I feel I am.

HIV disease is not something I have but something I am. I am HIV disease. However, I am more than that. I am also a thinking, caring, loving, hopeful person. I am always more than the existing feeling. I am more than anxious, for example. I am also courageous. The more aware I become of the feelings which coexist alongside the dominant or central feeling then the more able I become to select out that which I desire to become. When I allow my HIV disease to be the centre of who I am, I effectively surrender my potential to become anything else. Becoming better means that I give my other areas a chance to be actualised through action, through doing. At this very moment in time, for instance, I am a writer. I do not deny that I am other things also but I select out the writer. I become the writer. I am the writer. When I am fully occupied with writing I have no time or space to be anything else. To do this I must first stop doing everything else and listen to my inner self-potential. When I do this I give myself time to think and decide who I am to become.

LIVING WITH THE CENTRAL SELF

When I am alone with myself I can explore that which is to become a potential centre of who I am. The person who has the permanent centre of HIV disease may be unwilling, at this time, to take up the challenge it poses. He may be morbidly fixated and need reminding of those other things he is as well. There will, of course, be times when it is appropriate to make HIV disease the centre but even those times should come through choice.

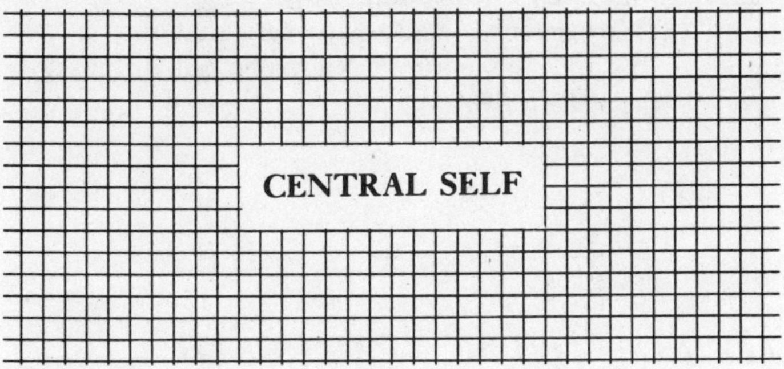

Selecting out that which is to be the centre of who I am is a positive act. It is not, however, an act which chooses who I am not. In choosing, I do not deny my other aspects. What I do is to give prominence to the centre. Before being able to do so, however, I must unload all unwanted baggage from my mind. I must 'go through' whatever amount of grief is called for. I must have allowed myself to have experienced all those things which demand attention. I must not rush at it. I must be patient and be prepared to take a step or two in other directions before moving forward again.

LIVING WITH THE PAST

How I determine the centre now will have major consequences not only on my future but also on my past. It will influence and filter in a way which will directly affect what and how I recall. When I am happy, for example, I tend to recall happy events. When I am depressed I tend to recall old suicide thoughts. The important thing for me to be aware of is that I am in a constant process of becoming. No matter what I do, I will become. Why not, therefore, become through conscious choice? Kierkegaard called this 'choosing one's self'. In so doing the person takes responsibility for his existence. Rollo May said that this is 'the opposite to blind momentum'. Nietzsche called the same process 'the will to live'.

LIVING WITH MENTAL DEATH

To take responsibility for my life means that I must become aware that I can end it. I can kill myself.

Not only can people kill themselves physically, they can kill themselves psychologically too. That is, a person, without even being aware of it, can choose not to live. He gives up his life through his will to die. What may be going on here is that he has made some negative aspect of himself the centre and that's what he is giving up because it is too painful to cope with. Helping him move his centre, by a reminder of his other aspects, may save his life.

Not only can individuals kill themselves mentally,

various groups in society can also inflict a kind of mental death on people with HIV disease. These are the groups who tend to see those with the disease as not worthy of looking after because 'they are going to die anyway'. They would have us go off somewhere and die quietly, without fuss. Caring people everywhere should respond to such rejection with justifiable anger. The time is perhaps right for us to not only have peaceful candle-lit vigils but also angry demonstrations each time a person dies from this disease. We should not delude ourselves that enough is being done!

LIVING WITH SELF-ELECTED DEATH

The saving of life is generally thought of as being something good and the ending of it, through suicide, as something bad. But is it? In the will to live there is an acknowledgement of, not the quantity, but the quality of life. When a person with HIV disease gets to the point when death is the known outcome, does that person not have the right, the responsibility even, to think and act on the quality of his death?

Helping people to die is not a new phenomenon. Good doctors have been helping people to die for generations. But is this, in the age of HIV disease, something that should be left to doctors alone? I think not. On my mother's death certificate it reads that she died of cancer. In fact she died of an ever-increasing drugs overdose, and all those who loved her were grateful to the compassion of her doctor in his efforts to prevent her experiencing avoidable pain. The doctor talked to us as family and we were fully aware of what was going on.

I know two men who have an agreement to help each other die at a given stage. They are a couple who love each other very much. Both have HIV disease and they are both aware of where that might take them. I respect their maturity greatly in being able to arrive at their decision in the light of the pressures of others' beliefs and attitudes.

'Suicide' is not the term which actively fits what these men have planned. Not least, because of the negative connotations inherent in the word. Sad, anxious and depressed people are the people who engage in 'suicide'. Euthanasia is not a suitable word either for it tends to imply the mercy of one person towards another. In this sense, my mother's death was euthanasia. 'Self-Elected Death' is a much more accurate term. It is thought through long before the event. It is planned in advance and deals with the notion of death in the term itself. It is more realistic.

Self-Elected Death is something which counsellors and others in the caring world should help drag out of the taboo closet in which it has been locked up for years. Paradoxically, the keepers of the keys here are those absolutists who force their morality, either knowingly or unknowingly, onto others. Those who do so unknowingly are often the most dedicated gaolers. Self-Elected Death is a reality we shall have to address sooner or later. If for no other reason than because of the numbers who select it as a choice and make that choice publicly known.

LIVING WITH MY DEATH

Without doubt one of the most vital issues to emerge out of my diagnosis has been that of death. It has come home to me that:

1. Death is almost a taboo subject;
2. Friends have great difficulty in talking about it;
3. Not many people prepare for death;

4. I can prepare for my death;
5. As a humanist, death is the end;
6. It is the loss of life which is sad, not death;
7. I need to initiate the grieving process myself;
8. I can decide when and how I die;
9. The knowledge of death enriches my life;
10. I alone must face my death.

The knowledge that I will die, and the challenge I face as a result, is to accept the creative opportunity to:

1. Put my life in order;
2. Do those things I've always wanted to do;
3. Draw up a list of priorities;
4. Say goodbye to loved ones;
5. Stop doing those things which are negative;
6. Write a detailed last will;
7. Design my funeral service;
8. Plan what is to become of my ashes;
9. Initiate grieving;
10. Select my place of death.

In the experience of accepting my death I discover that my drive to live a more creative and productive life is strengthened. I feel pushed to accomplish more. I become that much more alive. There is a strong spur for me to make something of my life. At the centre, at the moment, is the writer. The following piece of writing is a result:

A Humanistic Version of the 23rd Psalm

I am myself, I know this truth.
I reflect upon this and see my potential in the
reflection.
I am the screen on which I vision self.
I find serenity and calmness in this knowledge.
Even though there is no knowing I fear not
death,
For the unknown holds no fears.
The harmony of self with other is my guide.
I am nourished in doing what I am becoming.
My cup of love overfloweth through choice,
For I will live to my death and prepare for the
end.

Accepting my death does not mean that I want to die. Far from it. I want to live. More than that, I want to live a life long enough to do all the things I've ever dreamt of.

Tarry a while, O Death, I cannot die
With all my blossoming hopes unharvested,
My joys ungarnered, all my songs unsung,
And all my tears unshed.

Tarry a while, till I am satisfied
Of love and grief, of earth and altering sky;
Till all my human hungers are fulfilled,
O Death, I cannot die!

Sarojini Naidu.

LIVING WITH QUALITY

We British don't like to speak of death, let alone further the notion of a self-actualised death. That is, a death for which we are ready. HIV disease may change that, however.

More than any other disease before it HIV disease is not solely the concern of the medical profession. It is as much a psychological or a sociological issue as it is medical.

Being ready for death is being ready to enhance freedom, for the person who has learnt how to die has unlearnt how to be a slave. Knowing how to die frees us from all oppression and chains. Learning how to die is to learn how to live more fully. Living a fully human existence is not something which can be measured by time. Living is not a matter of how many years I live but of how I use my life. It is about quality not quantity. Some people live long lives and yet never really live at all. When we attempt to banish thoughts of death from conscious awareness we adversely affect the quality of our lives. The feelings attached to death will emerge in other ways, usually in anxiety. Repressing thoughts of death uses up vast stores of energy which might be better used to improve the quality of our existence.

LIVING WITH ASSERTION

To creatively disobey means that the new 'I' must be that much more assertive. The assertive person is open and flexible, genuinely concerned with the rights of others, yet at the same time able to establish very well his own rights.

Each of us should be able to choose for ourselves how we act and react. However, I for one have difficulty in saying and meaning 'no'. My British politeness is too well developed for my own good. What happens then is that I bottle things up and because the bottle can only hold so much, it tends to burst with aggressive frustration and I hurt other people. These contrasting modes of behaviour are identified like this:

BEHAVIOUR	RESULT
Non-assertive	Denying one's own rights
Aggressive	Denying the rights of others
Assertive	Acknowledging your rights and others' too

Being assertive is not being aggressive, bossy or domineering. 'Assertive behaviour is open, honest, non-manipulative, and involves the direct expression of one's feelings, preferences, needs or opinions in a manner that is neither threatening nor punishing towards the other person.' (Cooper, 1982).

Imagine this scene: You have HIV disease and have just started doing some voluntary work for a worthwhile organisation. You've indicated that you are willing to do anything to help. It's 4.30 pm and you usually finish at 4. In fact you've agreed to meet a friend at five o'clock to go to the cinema, and you're feeling a bit under the weather. The volunteer co-ordinator rushes in waving some papers. He has just had a telephone call from someone willing to give money to the project but some work needs doing on them 'right away!' You realise the work will take at least an hour. What do you do?

NON-ASSERTIVE RESPONSE: 'That's fine, leave them with me, I'll drop everything and attend to it right away.'

AGGRESSIVE RESPONSE: 'What the hell do you take me for? Do you think I've got nothing else to do in my life other than jump each time you call? What did your last slave die of?'

ASSERTIVE RESPONSE: 'I know it's important that this be done as soon as possible but I've made arrangements to meet a friend at five o'clock and I'm not feeling very well, so I can't do it now. However, I'll do it first thing tomorrow.'

Creative assertive behaviour allows me to cooperate, communicate and interact more effectively with others and at the same time to feel okay about myself.

Test your own level of assertion on the self-assessment table.

SELF-ASSESSMENT ASSERTION TABLE

HOW TO SCORE: To measure your assertiveness in each activity ask yourself, 'To what extent do I feel comfortable carrying out this activity with this person?' Put a tick in the appropriate box if your answer is yes.

	VARIOUS PEOPLE									
KINDS OF ACTIVITY	**1**	**2**	**3**	**4**	**5**	**6**	**7**	**8**	**9**	**10**
Expressing positive feelings; giving compliments										
Receiving compliments										
Express liking, love and affection										
Making requests, e.g. ask for favours, help, etc.										
Touch affectionately										
Initiate and maintain conversation about HIV										
Self-affirmation, stand up for your legitimate rights										
Refuse requests										
Refuse invitations										
Express personal opinions including disagreement										
Expressing negative feelings; express justified annoyance and displeasure										
Express justified anger										

NUMBERS CODE: 1 = Friends; 2 = Gay friends; 3 = Nurses; 4 = Doctor; 5 = Officials; 6 = Partner/s; 7 = Shop assistants; 8 = Co-workers; 9 = People with HIV disease; 10 = People without HIV disease.

LIVING WITH PARASITES

Being assertive also means that I must learn to be selective. It means I must choose sides and become an involved revolutionary. In the war being waged against HIV disease there are two fronts to the fight: the first is the fight to find a cure, the other is the fight carried out by those living with the disease to live as fully as possible. In this war there are only two sides, the side which aligns itself with those who have the disease and the side which doesn't. Not to align oneself with those who have the disease is to acquiesce with the other side. However, there are those who appear to be on the aligned side but are actually on the other. These are the parasitic moral saboteurs. They are the people who help for a price, yet may never appear to demand it, for the price they demand is the gratification of their own inner needs. Such people abuse the weakness of others to gain a position of strength for themselves. These are the people who appear to be doing one thing and are, in reality, doing something else. They are the people who open hospices for those with the disease where the aim is to deceptively sell their own religious beliefs. Such people are a menace and should be treated as such. With real caring there is never a disguised or an undisguised price to pay. Such people would do well to read Fr Bill Kirkpatrick's book *AIDS: Sharing the Pain*, published by Dartman, Longman & Todd, 1988. There speaks a true and sincere Christian whom I acknowledge from my own atheism.

LIVING WITH MORAL PROJECTIONS

Being assertive means that I must reject both the disguised and undisguised moral projections of others. As a Gay man with HIV disease this is more important than ever before. Not least, to counter the charge that Gay men are themselves responsible for the existence of the disease. Not only is this charge without foundation but it also effectively denies the enormous efforts which Gay men have made to prevent the spread of the disease. I am proud to be associated with an international Gay community which has achieved so much in the field of caring responsibility.

Moral projections come in all shapes and sizes but all have one thing in common. Namely, that the nature of the projection says more about the persons doing the projecting than it does about the person or group onto whom the projection is focused.

Morally projected identifications work in this way:

A person, usually through lack of knowledge and for reasons often related to his own inner moral fears, will perceive a phenomenon in purely moral terms. That is, as being either good or bad. In so doing he has little time to consider the actual nature of the phenomenon. Not only does he not have time but he also, through the internal processes of repression and denial, actively prevents himself from making the time. To address the nature of the phenomenon would be too difficult for him. Not least, because he may be forced to reconsider his position in relation to it. By closing his mind to the nature of the phenomenon and concentrating instead on his own moral opinions of it, he effectively escapes having to think it through. His 'achievement', therefore, is to distance himself from the confronting phenomenon. When he judges the phenomenon as being bad, homosexuality for instance, he then goes one stage further and assumes the homosexual person to be bad also. His logic being that if homosexuality is bad therefore those who indulge in it are bad for so doing. Because he has a closed mind he is likely to look into any work, the Bible for instance, to confirm his views. In so doing he is confirmed in his opinions. Psychologically he cannot lose, but in truth he cannot win.

Such a person can never know the value to be had in friendship, for he will always be on his guard and ready only to offer a censored self to his censured projections. When such a man says 'yes' to something the chances are that he will have no idea why he's saying 'no' to the opposite. In his moral absolutist position he will fail to see that the greatest knowledge is that he'll never know and that there is no easy road to truth. When this man condemns homosexuals for their sexuality he assumes the homosexual to have chosen his orientation, and because none of us homosexuals are permanently or continuously good he finds moral justification in the elements of truth he sees from his narrowed position.

Such a person is capable only of offering sympathy from a superior position. He can know nothing of empathy. That is, he does not have the capacity to imaginatively share the feeling, ideas or identity of another person outside of himself.

In contrast, however, my empathetic friend sees the unique mystery that is me. Never fully understanding it nor too deeply exploring it, he allows it to be. He sees this mystery and knows it to be the evolving me. He sees and knows that it's mine and mine alone. He sees the possibilities for growth and allows it to happen. Sometimes the results please him, sometimes not. He sees the mystery that is me and lets it be, for me, for others and for himself. He sees me as a whole person. Not always complete and together, nor loose and lost. He sees the whole me and accepts this wholeness. This indeed makes him my friend. He sees the strengths and weaknesses, the potential and limitations, the clear views and the blockages, the caring and the selfishness, the harmony and the discord, the saint and the sinner. He sees it all and accepts. He sees the struggle and the ease of my move towards change and the greater me, and allows it to happen at my pace. He sometimes sees just how slow it is and how many backward steps I have to retrace in an effort to get it right in my own terms. He sees me as a person who knows the value of true friendship but also as a person who sometimes lets him down. He is safe in the knowledge that I would never knowingly hurt him. So when I do, the process of healing is co-creative. He knows that I'll try to dwell more on the recovery than on the hurt itself. He sees that in wounding I'm wounded too. He sees the sensitivity that is in me and is careful to encourage and preserve it. But he also sees the times when I'm just a little too introspective and self-centred and he makes allowances. He sees the person who needs loving, who wants to give, who needs to be needed, the searcher after truth, the child and the adult, the poet and the writer, the Marxist who reads the Bible, the guy who says he wants a lot of new experiences but who is often just too lazy to move. My friend sees the paradox that is me and my efforts to work it through constructively. He sees the aggression and the frustration and my efforts to cope with such powerful energy. He sees me growing through trying. He sees my HIV disease and does not make it the centre of his or my world. His seeing helps me see myself so much more honestly. The strength of his growing acceptance of the total me permits me to be growingly vulnerable towards him, so allowing myself to see myself as I am through his eyes. His 'seeing' and my acceptance of it allows the mystery that is me to remain intact and free to evolve.

LIVING WITH EROTIC SEX

The first thing to be said about 'safer sexuality' is, if you haven't tried it, don't knock it. Erotic sexuality does not have to be unsafe to be good and very few of us have explored the full range of our sexual potential. Exploring the nature of our sexuality may bring remarkable results. Before we begin, however, we have to want to. We shouldn't force it or be pressed into doing it. We have to take our time. It might be wise to start alone. Be as sure as you can that you're not going to be disturbed and have a pen and paper handy. You won't need anything else at this stage. Now, turn to the Safer Sexuality table and look it over. This table can never be long enough, but list those things which come to mind without any order of priority. When you are ready, tick either the 'safe' or 'unsafe' boxes. Then go through the list and decide for yourself which of the unsafe can be made safer and how. If you don't know what is 'safe' or 'unsafe' go to the section on 'Living with Risk' first.

I hope to produce a book on 'Living With Safer Sex' quite soon.

SEXUAL LIKES	SAFE?	UNSAFE?	MAY BE MADE SAFER BY	OPTIONS?

PLEASE NOTE: FOR DETAILED ADVICE ON 'SAFER SEX', ON WHAT CONSTITUTES A 'RISK' AND WHETHER OR NOT A PARTICULAR SEXUAL ACT IS RISKY, CONTACT THE TERRENCE HIGGINS TRUST AT 52-54 GRAY'S INN ROAD, LONDON WC1X 8CT OR TELEPHONE THEIR HELPLINE ON 01-242 1010. IF IN DOUBT, ASK FOR ADVICE BEFORE DOING ANYTHING RISKY. REMEMBER, PREVENTION IS ALWAYS BETTER.

LIVING WITH RISKS

The risk of either passing on or picking up the HIV virus through sexual contact is very real, as is the risk of either passing on or picking up other sexually transmittable infections. Everyone who is sexually active is at risk. The exchange of 'cum' (semen) and 'pre-cum' should be avoided. The exchange of blood should be avoided. The use of either alcohol or poppers may impair your judgement and therefore compromise your immune system. This applies to all other drugs too. In both anal and vaginal intercourse use a condom. But remember, condoms can and sometimes do break during use.

SOME SEXUAL ALTERNATIVES:

1. Touching, caressing, massage. Try massaging each other absolutely everywhere. There is no risk whatsoever of passing on or picking up the virus this way. Massage oils are sold in 'Body Shops'. If you can't get massage oil try baby oil instead. Take showers and baths together and experiment. It's fun and it's SAFE!

2. Mutual masturbation. Wanking together or each other can often be a great deal more enjoyable than penetrative sex. Try sharing a fantasy or listening to your partner's fantasy. It's fun and it's SAFE!

3. Solo masturbation. This is an activity that most of us know something about already. If you don't then now is the time to find out. There is more than one way to masturbate. What about with massage oil? With a rubber on? Without hands? (Requires a bit of imagination, that one.) It's fun and it's SAFE!

4. Condoms. Don't use oil-based lubricants with condoms as they are that much more likely to break. Condoms should always be worn when you engage in either oral or penetrative sex. With oral sex try covering the condom (after it's on) with fresh cream and have your partner lick it off. Fill a condom with water and freeze it, then use it as a dildo. When your partner is wearing the condom try this: have your mouth full of something hot — like tea or coffee, and then try oral sex. Vary the something hot with something cold like fruit juice. It's fun and it's SAFE!

SAFER SEXUALITY REQUIRES IMAGINATION

Start at the square with the * in. Have fun!

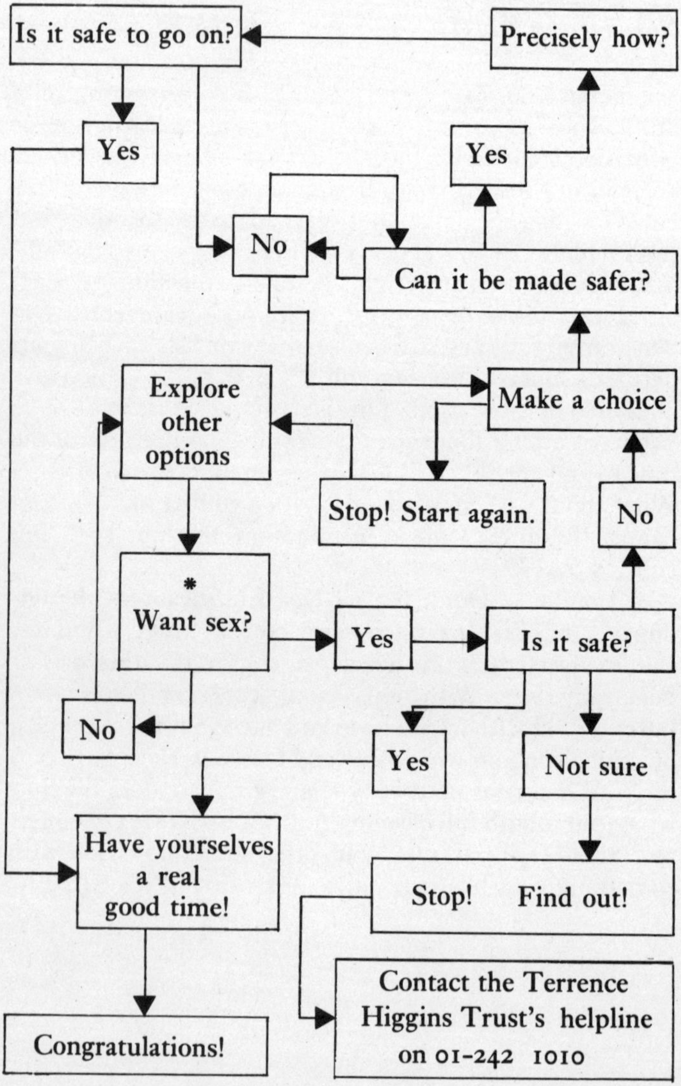

There are some distinct advantages to adopting a safer sexuality stance:

1. Better health;
2. More intimacy;
3. Dating;
4. Longer love-making sessions;
5. Affection;
6. More imagination;
7. Romance;
8. Less performance anxiety;
9. STD reduction;
10. More control;
11. More variety;
12. More love-making, less just having sex;
13. More talk and communication;
14. Greater realisation and actualisation of the full self.

15.

16.

17.

18.

19.

20.

SOME GENERAL GUIDELINES:

* Don't exchange body fluids, particularly semen (cum) and vaginal secretions.

* Don't have any kind of sex which is likely to break the skin or sensitive membranes. This means: no biting, no fisting, no rough or violent activity which you know from past experience causes small scratches or cuts.

* Don't engage in 'water sports' (pissing on each other).
* Don't go in for 'rimming' (oral stimulation of the anus).
* Don't go in for unprotected anal intercourse. The muscular tissue inside the anus tears very easily. Remember that CONDOMS DO BREAK!
* Don't come in your partner's mouth, or allow them to come in yours. Genital and mouth sores increase the likelihood of transmission.
* Don't try anything with your partner without their full informed consent.

In learning to adopt a 'new sexuality' I have to consider three things:

1. The loss of my pre-HIV sexuality. I should allow myself to mourn the loss just as often as I want to.
2. The discovery of my post-HIV sexuality. I should continue to explore options for as long as I want.
3. Learning to eroticise my new sexuality. I should experiment in ways which I feel comfortable with.

Imagine this scene: You're in a pub and the beautiful person you've had your eye on comes over to talk with you. You start to flirt with each other and it becomes clear that you both want to make love. How do you bring up the subject of safer sexuality?

NEGATIVELY: 'I really like you and I'm sorry to have to mention this but I'm into safer sex...'

POSITIVELY: 'Let's get out of here. I have a great safer sex idea I want to share with you...'

OR, BETTER STILL:

Your affirming confidence will help reduce the other person's possible embarrassment. If, however, the person is turned off by the notion of safer sexuality, then you've found out at the right time, haven't you?

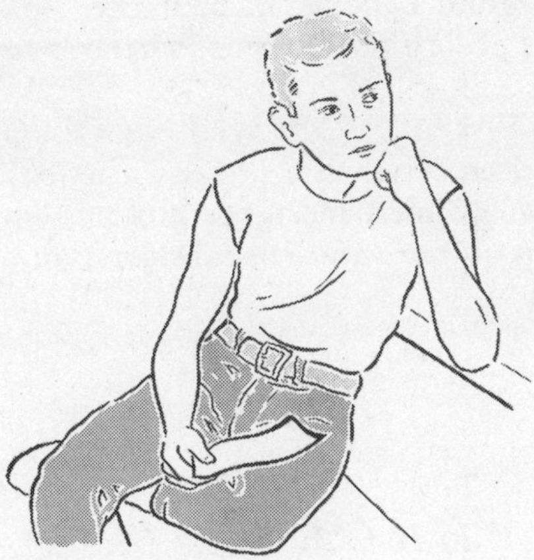

LIVING WITH THE TEST

There are good reasons both for and against taking the test and each person should decide for themselves. If you are unsure about these reasons then do contact the Terrence Higgins Trust and unashamedly ask for advice.

THE TEST.
Support and counselling may be required:

When thinking about taking the test;
Before taking the test;
After taking the test;
Before going for the results;
After getting the results;
When dealing with the results.

Support should involve the process of information giving and education. No two people will have the same knowledge or insight into HIV and we should never assume that the person understands the nature of the test or the workings of the virus. The test procedure should be explained both verbally and in writing, as should the outcome and consequences of being given either a negative or positive result. Time should be allowed for the person to emotionally absorb their results, whatever they are.

THERE IS NOTHING TO STOP ANYONE USING A FALSE NAME WHEN GOING FOR THE TEST! Indeed, given the present reactions from some insurance companies, mortgage brokers, employers and the like it is an option worth consideration.

LIVING WITH COUNSELLING

The humanist counsellor does not hold that the client is determined either by unconscious or learned behaviour patterns. In my own experience of learning to deal more effectively with HIV disease I know that there is that fleeting moment between stimulus and response when, through an act of choosing, I have discovered the authenticity of self-respect. From the high ground of self-respect I am able to be more authentically myself through self-enactment.

However, when I fail to listen attentively to the wisdom of selfhood I tune in, instead, to the values and attitudes of others in order that they may love and respect me more. In doing this I effectively give up my rights to self-determination. I allow others to dictate who I am. I cease to be the prime mover.

Even within the inner world of counselling there is no

one definition that satisfies the various practitioners. Look for example at the following five definitions and draw your own conclusions:

Counselling is:

1. 'The giving of advice on personal, social, psychological, etc. problems as an occupation.' (*Oxford English Dictionary*, 1972.)

2. 'A dialogue in which one person helps another who has some difficulty that is important to him.' (Wallis, 1973.)

3. 'A process designed to help a person answer the question "What shall I do". (Tyler, 1961.)

4. 'An enabling process, designed to help an individual to come to terms with his life as it is and ultimately to grow to greater maturity through learning to take responsibility and make decisions himself.' (Jones, 1970.)

5. 'The way in which a counsellor and his client relate to each other in the exploration together of the client's problem and possible solution to it. Counselling is generally differentiated from the treatment of patients; its basic orientation is not to psychopathology but to the types of problems people encounter at different stages of their normal human development.' (Thompson, 1970.)

It is worth dwelling on some of the key words in those definitions. 'Helps' and 'difficulty' in quote number two; 'help' in number three; 'help', 'come to terms', 'maturity' and 'responsibility' in number four; 'problem', 'normal' and 'psychopathology' in number five. All these words are value laden and may well lead one into going along with the drift of the definition without too much questioning. Yet it is these very words and phrases which must be questioned, for they either explain or disguise the true intent of the counsellor. I've selected out what are for me, at the time of writing, the key words. This is done not to suggest that they invariably are so but to draw our attention to the notion of semantics. Semantics is about meaning and when values are involved we are in danger of either being misunderstood or of misunderstanding,

So it is that I do not know what the writers of the five definitions mean by 'help' or the 'process' of helping. I think I know what I mean, but is that the same thing? I think not. Clearly then, when the client meets the counsellor two obvious assumptive worlds are at liberty and may collide. When I, the person with HIV disease, meet you, the person without the disease, we are in danger of missing each other completely. A major goal in counselling, therefore, must be to discover what is actually meant from the words selected to express the feeling. In HIV counselling, as in all good counselling, the more real and congruent the person doing the counselling is, is far more important than the theory he values. Indeed, he is likely to value a particular theory because of the person he is.

Because of these two assumptive worlds a false consciousness may emerge which could trap the counsellor into thinking that he is actually doing what he thinks he is doing. What we think we do and what we actually do may be different. When a person seeks counselling he may, in reality, be in search of something which isn't actually on offer. What he undertands counselling to be may not be the same as what the counsellor understands it to be. Counselling, if it is anything, should always be a search for meanings and can only really be defined each time it takes place. That is, its definition emerges out of the ontological context in which it is practised in the here and now experience.

Counsellors working in and around the HIV issue

achieve power through their knowledge and are, without insight into the nature of that power, in very real danger of becoming no more than agents of control on behalf of the agency or group they represent. Counselling skills may be used or abused both knowingly and unknowingly. The unknowing counsellor is likely to keep his client weak in order to make him dependent.

Objectivity in HIV counselling can only ever be a goal, for it is very rarely achieved. Each aspect of HIV disease has both its objective and its subjective features. There is HIV disease, that we know is an objective fact. However, what I know about the nature of HIV and how I relate that knowledge constitutes a subjective fact. How different people with HIV disease report honestly how they feel about their infection is a subjective fact. It may well be different from how others feel but as such it is correct. The counsellor's objectivity here is arrived at through his sensitive awareness of his client's views. The counsellor may have an objective intent but this is always subject to the forces of his client's existence as experienced at the time by the client.

An example of this could be as follows. Both counsellor and client are sitting together in the same room, on the wall is a thermometer that reads seventy degrees. The objective fact is that the room is seventy degrees. However, the client may feel cold whilst the counsellor feels too hot. Facts don't always speak for themselves, therefore. We should never assume we know anything about a client. We should constantly check things out first. A simple question, 'How do you feel about the room temperature?' might help. As John Powell points out in his book, *Why Am I Afraid To Tell You Who I Am*, 'If I am anything as a person, it is what I think, judge, feel, value, honour, esteem, love, hate, fear, desire, hope for, believe in and am committed to.'

BASIC HIV COUNSELLING CONSIDERATIONS:

1. Shock: No person is ever 'ready' for the news that he is infected with HIV.

2. The unknown: A person given a positive result will have a great many 'unknowns' to deal with. Not least, the possibility of going on to develop AIDS, the changes to be made in living patterns and so on.

3. Anxiety and depression: These conditions may be experienced as either slight or as quite overwhelming.

4. Loss and grief: Accepting the diagnosis means having to let go of previous sexual patterns. That alone is worth grieving about.

5. Making adjustments: Changing is not an easy process.

6. Retaining self-control: The person may not feel 'in control' of his life.

7. Guilt: The person may feel guilty about how he contracted the infection.

8. Relationships: Maintaining and making new relationships may prove to be quite difficult.

9. Isolation: The person might cut himself off from all contacts or may fear that others will cut him off.

10. Death: Some people want to talk about it, some don't. Some have little fear of death itself but a huge fear about the process of dying.

There are other considerations and I urge you to list just three more:

1.

2.

3.

LIVING WITH THE DOLE AND DHSS

People who have to give up their work should consider a number of issues:

1. Talk this through with your doctor first. If he agrees that it would be better for you to give up your present job, then ask him to supply you with a letter stating that you are not able to continue in the job because of your HIV disease.

2. Write to your employers telling them why you are leaving and keep a copy of the letter. You writing to them ensures that you get a letter back — which you'll need when it comes to claiming benefits.

3. Make a number of photocopies of the letters. You may need these for the Unemployment Benefit office and the DHSS. Don't send anything other than copies. Keep the originals. You may need them again.

4. If you leave your job without just cause you will not get any benefits for 13 weeks. That letter from your doctor gives you 'just cause'. The Unemployment office will contact your last employer to check out that what you have told them is the truth. That's why you had to have an answer in writing!

5. If you intend to make yourself available for further work be careful when filling in the forms you will be given, or sent, by the Department of Employment. Make it clear on those forms that you are prepared to consider any other work other than the your usual work. Not to do so could result in your not being given unemployment benefit because of your lack of availability. Also make it clear that you don't mind reasonable travelling. What you actually do later is your affair.

6. If you are too ill to take on another job like the one you've just given up, it might be in your financial interest to

tell both the Department of Employment and the DHSS that you are looking for a less stressful job. Not least, because Unemployment Benefit may be higher than Sickness payments.

7. When you go to the Unemployment Benefit office to 'sign on', don't be put off by the experience, and don't forget to take the photocopies of the letters with you. Take a pen along too. You are there to get money. Be quietly patient, you may have to wait around for quite some time. Take a book with you. Take your doctor's letter with you. Don't leave without a form B1. This you fill in and send to the DHSS, which is how you claim Supplementary Benefits.

If you are unsure about what you can and can't claim then contact the Terrence Higgins Trust and ask for help. If you live in the London area telephone the DHSS freephone number and ask for advice. You do this by dialing 100 and asking for the DHSS freephone. This won't cost you anything. Dotted around the country are advice centres which can be of great help. Check with the information section at the local Town Hall or with the Social Services department. In some areas now there are AIDS liaison workers who can be most helpful. Again, ask at your Town Hall.

NEED A FREE HOLIDAY?

If you haven't had a holiday for two years or more, and you are claiming benefits, contact the Social Work Department of the hospital you attend and ask them to contact the Percy Bilton Charity on your behalf on 01-579 2829. You cannot apply directly yourself. Requests must go through the hospital social work unit. The Percy Bilton Charity can provide a holiday for you in this country.

OTHER GRANTS: Try looking through the following books in your local Reference Library:

A Guide to the Major Grant-Making Trusts, edited by Luke Fitzherbert. Published by The Directory of Social Change, Radius Works, Back Lane, London, NW3 1HL (tel. 01-435 8171). Price £12.50.

A Guide to Grants for Individuals in Need, edited by Luke Fitzherbert and Helene Bellofatto. A Directory of Social Change publication. Price £9.95.

Directory of Grant-Making Trusts. Published by Charities Aid Foundation, 48 Pembury Road, Tonbridge, Kent, TN9 2JD. Price £45.00.

LIVING WITH ENHANCEMENT

Abraham H. Maslow pioneered a psychology of optimism which pointed to the inherent goodness in people. A human being is not a 'lump of clay' but has an essence which searches for actualisation. He concluded that what you can be, you must be, and that you have a 'hierarchy of basic needs' which almost automatically direct your life. After the gratification of hunger, which is the most basic of needs, you seek to gratify your need for feelings of safety, belongingness, love and self-esteem, more or less in that order. The need to be self-actualising, that is, to let your self guide your life, ranks just after these.

The Self-Actualising person tends to be:

* Emotionally 'grown up' to his full height;
* Brilliantly alive, alert and radiant;
* In touch with reality;
* More perceptive and accepting of himself and others;
* Unconventional and spontaneous without fuss;
* Rarely conforms for conformity's sake;

* Creatively disobedient, but not for its own sake;
* Able to receive satisfaction from within;
* Able to enjoy solitude;
* Self-directed;
* Free of needs to impress others;
* Able to enjoy sexuality;
* Able to accept death.

There is absolutely no reason in the world why a person with HIV disease should not start on a path to self-actualisation. Indeed, to do so will enhance his life greatly. So how does one go about it? Here, paraphrased from a talk given by Maslow (by Lewis & Streitfeld in their book *Growth Games*), are eight modest beginnings:

1. DEVOTE YOURSELF TOTALLY TO EXPERIENCING ONE MOMENT.
Try to feel it fully and unselfconsciously, the way a child would. Become totally absorbed in it, to the exclusion of everything else. You probably have such moments of intense concentration occasionally; you can make them happen more frequently. 'At this moment of experiencing,' noted Malsow, 'the person is wholly and fully human....This is a moment when the self is actualising itself.'

2. THINK OF LIFE AS A 'PROCESS OF CHOICES, ONE AFTER ANOTHER'.
You have to make dozens of choices a day. Each time, you decide either to progress or regress; to move on in development or to fall back on habit and fear. Try to make the growth choice more and more. 'Self-actualisation,' according to Maslow, 'is an ongoing process.' If you make the growth choice instead of the fear choice a dozen times a day, you thus 'move a dozen times a day towards self-actualisation.'

3. LISTEN TO THE 'IMPULSE VOICES' INSIDE YOUR SELF.

Look within your self for your tastes and decisions. 'Most of us,' Maslow pointed out, 'listen not to ourselves but to Mommy's introjected voice or Daddy's voice or to the voice of the Establishment, of the Elders, of authority, or of tradition.' Concentrate instead on how you actually feel about something, not how you think you are expected to feel.

4. WHEN IN DOUBT, BE HONEST RATHER THAN NOT.

Most of us opt for diplomacy and discretion, rather than honesty, when we're in doubt about what to say. But if you are honest, you are looking to your self for answers, and you are taking responsibility for what you find in yourself. And each time you take responsibility for yourself, you are taking a step towards actualising your self.

5. BE COURAGEOUS.

Dare to be different. Risk making unpopular statements if they reflect what you feel. In the avant-garde art world, Maslow feels, a conformity of taste is demanded. Most people try to make sophisticated-sounding remarks about the art they don't understand. Instead, be prepared to say, 'I don't know what to make of that dance programme. I'll have to think about it.' Or, 'That painting puzzles me.'

6. FIND OUT WHAT YOU WANT TO DO, AND WORK HARD TO DO IT WELL.

Be as first-rate as you can. This may mean, says Maslow, going through an arduous period of preparation to realise your possibilities.

7. LEAVE YOURSELF OPEN TO PEAK EXPERIENCES, THOSE 'LITTLE MOMENTS OF ECSTACY' — FOR THEY ARE FLEETING MOMENTS OF SELF-ACTUALISATION.
Try to set up conditions in which peak experiences are more likely to occur, and accept them when they do. According to Maslow, almost everyone has peak experiences, but 'some people wave these small mystical experiences aside' and deny them. Instead, look for them, and savour them.

8. AS MUCH AS POSSIBLE, IDENTIFY YOUR DEFENCES.
That is, behaviour patterns you have seized upon to protect you from emotional pain. Find the courage to give them up. This is painful but necessary, for repressing a problem won't solve it.

LIVING WITH MEDITATIONS

Allowing yourself just a short time each day to be alone with yourself can greatly improve the quality of your life. Here is a meditation you might care to try. Read it through first before finding a quiet space. Try lying down with a small cushion supporting your neck. Start by making every muscle in your body tight — then let go.

THE JOINING

Close your eyes.

Hear the name of the one you love...
Let it echo within...

That name alone...
Over and over...
Fills you.

Listen to the name...
Melting into you...
Becoming you...

Frontiers of self...
Moving to it...

Breathe in the name...
Breathe out the joining.

Let the muscles of your face relax...
to the joining...

Only the name repeats itself...
Relax...
Let go...

LIVING WITH SELF-AWARENESS

How much do you know about yourself? Living with self-awareness is also about living with self-disclosure and sharing. Here is an invitation to an experiment. You can try this alone, with a soul-friend or in a group. Below is a window with six panes. Fill in each pane as accurately as you can right away. Then, do some sensitive research with your soul friend or group and have another go at filling in the panes. You could try asking the other to fill in pane number 2 for you. This can be very revealing and requires mutual trust.

Things that others know (about me) 1	Things others know and I don't know (about me) 2
Things I know others don't know (about me) 3	Things no one knows (about me) 4
Things I might consider sharing with others (about me) 5	Things I will share (about me) with others 6

A variation of that window is:

Things others know about my HIV. 1	Things others know and I don't know about my HIV. 2
Things I know others don't know about my HIV. 3	Things no one knows about my HIV. 4
Things I might consider sharing about my HIV. 5	Things I will share with selected others about my HIV. 6

FURTHER INFORMATION

TERRENCE HIGGINS TRUST
BM/AIDS, London WC1N 3XX
Telephone: 01-242 1010 (Mon-Fri 7pm to 10pm, Sat & Sun 3pm to 10pm)

BODY POSITIVE
P.O. Box 493, London W14 0TF

NATIONAL ADVISORY SERVICE ON AIDS
Telephone: 0800-567 123 (10am to 10pm)

GAY SWITCHBOARD
BM Switchboard, London WC1N 3XX
Telephone: 01-837 7324

HAEMOPHILIA SOCIETY
123 Westminster Bridge Road, London SE1 7HR
Telephone: 01-428 2020

SCODA (Standing Committe on Drug Abuse)
1-4 Hatton Place, London EC1N 8ND
Telephone: 0430-2341

HEALTH EDUCATION AUTHORITY
78 New Oxford Street, London WC1
Telephone: 01-631 0930

REFERENCES AND BIBLIOGRAPHY

Allport, Gordon, W., *Becoming: Basic Considerations for a Psychology of Personality*, Yale University Press, 1955.

Arieti, Silvano, *Creativity: The Magic Synthesis*, Basic Books, New York, 1976.

Cooper, C. L., 'Coping With Stress After Sensitivity Training', *Psychological Reports*, 1972, 31, 602.

Cooper, C. L., *Improving Interpersonal Relations*, Prentice-Hall, Engelwood Cliffs, New Jersey, 1982.

De Mello, Anthony, *Wellsprings: A Book of Spirtual Exercises*, Gujarat Sahitya Prakash, Anand, India, 1984.

Frankl, Victor E., *Man's Search for Meaning*, London, 1984.

Fromm, Erich, *On Disobedience and Other Essays*, London 1984.

Fromm, Erich, *The Fear of Freedom*, London, 1960.

Fromm, Erich, *To Have Or To Be*, London, 1978.

Fromm, Erich, *The Sane Society*, London, 1956.

Fromm, Erich, *The Art of Loving*,London, 1976.

Fromm, Erich, *Beyond the Chains of Illusion*, London, 1980.

Goodman, Lisl M., *Death and the Creative Life*, Springer Publishing Company, New York, 1976.

Goodman, Marburg L., *Attitudes Towards Death as a Function of Age and Level of Accomplishment*, 21st International Congress of Psychology, Paris, 1976.

Heidegger, Martin, *The Question of Being*, College & University Press, New Haven, USA, 1958.

Hewitt, James, *Relaxation East and West: A Manual of Poised Living*, London, 1982.

Jones, Anne, *School Counselling in Practice*, London, 1970.

Kaufmann, Walter, *Existentialism, Religion and Death*, New American Library, New York, 1976.

Kirkpatrick, Fr. Bill, *AIDS: Sharing the Pain*, London, 1988.

Lewis, H. R., & Streitfeld, H. S., *Growth Games*, London, 1972.

May, Rollo, *The Discovery of Being: Writings in Existential Psychology*, London, 1983.

May, Rollo, *Man's Search for Himself*, London, 1975.

Mayeroff, Milton, *On Caring*, Perennial Library, Harper & Row, New York, 1971.

Merton, Thomas, *No Man Is an Island*, London, 1955.

Montaigne, Michel de, *That To Philosophise Is To Learn To Die, The Complete Essays of Montaigne*, Stanford University Press, Palo Alto, California, 1965.

Osborne, A. F., *Applied Imagination*, Scribner's, New York, 1953.

Parad, Howard, *Crisis Intervention: Selected Readings*, Family Services Association of America, 1965.

Rossman, Joseph, *The Psychology of the Inventor*, Inventors Publishers, New York, 1931.

Stein, M. I., 'Creativity and Culture', in Mooney, R. L., & Razik, T. A. (eds), *Explorations in Creativity*, Harper & Row, New York, 1967.

Stein, M. I., *Stimulating Creativity, Vol. 1: Individual Procedures*,Academic Press, New York, 1974.

Storr, Anthony, *The Dynamics of Creation*, 1972.

Taylor, C. W., Berry, P. C., & Block, C. H., 'Does Group Participation When Using Brainstorming Facilitate or Inhibit Creative Thinking', ONR Technical Memorandum, Psychology Department, Yale University, 1957.

Tepl, Johannes von, *Der Ackermann und der Tod*, Insel-Verlag, Weisbaden, 1400.

Thompson, A. J. M., *An Investigation into the Work Performed by Some Trained Counsellors in English Secondary Schools*, Keele, 1970.

Tyler, Leona, *The Work of the Counsellor*, London, 1961.

Vinacke, W. E., *The Psychology of Thinking*, McGraw-Hill, New York, 1952.

Wallas, Joseph, *The Art of Thought*, Harcourt, Brace, New York, 1926.

Wright, Derek, *The Psychology of Moral Behaviour*, Harmondsworth, 1971.